# EAT TO BEAT
# YOUR
# DIET

## RECIPES BOOK

20 Diet Solution To Activate Your Body, Burn Fat Naturally And Heal Your Metabolism To Lose Weight Easily.

## MARIYAM MOHL

### EAT TO BEAT YOUR DIET RECIPES BOOK

## Copyright © 2023 by Mariyam Mohl

All rights reserved. No part of this publication may be reproduced, distributed, or transmitted in any form or by any means, including photocopying, recording, or other electronic or mechanical methods, without the prior written permission of the publisher, except in the case of brief quotations embodied in critical reviews and certain other noncommercial uses permitted by copyright law.

EAT TO BEAT YOUR DIET RECIPES BOOK

# TABLE OF CONTENT

INTRODUCTION ........................................... 5
   Baked Apples with Cinnamon and Walnuts .. 7
   Cabbage and Lentil Soup ......................... 10
   Blackened Tilapia Tacos with Cabbage Slaw
   ........................................................... 13
   Mango and Chicken Lettuce Wraps ........... 16
   Zucchini Noodles with Pesto and Cherry
   Tomatoes .............................................. 19
   Kale and Quinoa Stuffed Bell Peppers ....... 22
   Egg White Omelette with Spinach and Feta 25
   Turkey and Vegetable Lettuce Wraps ........ 28
   Cauliflower Pizza with Veggie Toppings ..... 31
   Greek Yogurt Parfait with Fresh Berries ..... 35
   Recipe: Spaghetti Squash with Turkey
   Bolognese ............................................. 38
   Vegetarian Stir-Fry with Tofu and Broccoli . 41
   Quinoa Salad with Mixed Vegetables and
   Lemon Vinaigrette .................................. 44
   Chickpea and Spinach Curry .................... 47
   Salmon and Asparagus Foil Packets .......... 50
   Turkey and Vegetable Skewers with Greek
   Yogurt Sauce ......................................... 53
   Shrimp and Avocado Salad ...................... 56

# EAT TO BEAT YOUR DIET RECIPES BOOK

Baked Cod with Lemon and Dill................ 59
Sweet Potato and Black Bean Enchiladas... 62
Grilled Chicken Breast with Herb Marinade 66
CONCLUSION ........................................... 69

# INTRODUCTION

Welcome to the "Eat to Beat Your Diet Recipes Book," a compilation of recipes created with the science of weight loss in mind. This culinary adventure is intended to not only help you achieve your dietary objectives but to exceed them. With the help of this book, we'll go on a delectable culinary adventure and discover dishes that will help you on your path to become a better and more fit version of yourself.

This collection's basic tenet is to nourish your body with full, nutrient-dense foods and allow the delectable flavors to add delight to your weight loss quest.

The days of boring and constrictive diets are long gone, and one recipe at a time, we think that taking care of your health can be enjoyable.

You'll find a selection of recipes in these pages that have been thoughtfully chosen to support your weight loss goals. Every recipe on this page, from colorful salads full of fresh fruit to filling main courses full of lean proteins and whole grains, is proof that you don't have to give up flavor to reach your fitness and health objectives.

# EAT TO BEAT YOUR DIET RECIPES BOOK

The "Eat to Beat Your Diet Recipes Book" has a wide range of recipes that highlight the splendor of a well-balanced diet. These recipes are designed to be easy and accessible for all skill levels, whether you are an experienced home cook or you are just getting started.

To help you along the way, there are clear directions, eye-catching pictures, and—above all—a breakdown of the nutritional advantages of each recipe.

However, this book serves as more than just a recipe book—rather, it's a guide for adopting a healthy way of life. In addition to the delicious recipes, you'll learn about the nutritional advantages of important components, practical advice on mindful eating, and a manual for creating long-lasting routines that support your weight loss objectives.

Now let's flip the page and enter a world where flavor and nutrition are complementary. The "Eat to Beat Your Diet Recipes Book" is more than simply a recipe book; it's a call to rethink how you relate to food and adopt a lifestyle in which each meal is a step toward a happier, healthier you.

Toast to tasty discoveries and the path to overcoming your diet!

# EAT TO BEAT YOUR DIET RECIPES BOOK

## Baked Apples with Cinnamon and Walnuts

**Ingredients:**
- 4 medium-sized apples (such as Honeycrisp or Granny Smith)
- 1/4 cup chopped walnuts
- 2 tablespoons honey or maple syrup
- 1 teaspoon ground cinnamon
- 1 tablespoon unsalted butter, cut into small pieces
- Pinch of salt

**Instructions:**
1. **Preheat the Oven:**
   - Preheat your oven to 375°F (190°C).
2. **Prepare the Apples:**
   - Wash and core the apples, leaving the bottoms intact to create a well for the filling.
3. **Prepare the Filling:**
   - In a small bowl, mix together the chopped walnuts, honey (or maple syrup), ground cinnamon, and a pinch of salt.

4. **Fill the Apples:**
    - Stuff each cored apple with the walnut mixture, pressing it down gently.
5. **Top with Butter:**
    - Place a small piece of butter on top of each filled apple.
6. **Bake:**
    - Arrange the stuffed apples in a baking dish and bake in the preheated oven for 25-30 minutes or until the apples are tender.
7. **Baste with Juices:**
    - Periodically baste the apples with the juices from the bottom of the baking dish to keep them moist.
8. **Serve Warm:**
    - Remove from the oven and let the apples cool for a few minutes before serving. Optionally, drizzle with additional honey or maple syrup.

**Benefits:**
1. **Rich in Fiber:** Apples are a great source of dietary fiber, promoting digestive health and helping you feel full.
2. **Healthy Fats:** Walnuts contribute heart-healthy omega-3 fatty acids.
3. **Natural Sweetness:** Honey or maple syrup provides sweetness without refined sugars.

4. **Antioxidants:** Cinnamon is loaded with antioxidants that may have anti-inflammatory effects.
5. **Vitamins and Minerals:** Apples and walnuts provide essential vitamins and minerals, including vitamin C and potassium.

**Application:**
- **Dessert:** Serve as a wholesome dessert, either on its own or with a dollop of Greek yogurt for added creaminess.
- **Breakfast:** Enjoy baked apples as a nutritious breakfast option, paired with a side of protein like yogurt or cottage cheese.
- **Snack:** Satisfy your sweet tooth with a baked apple as a satisfying and nutritious snack.

## Cabbage and Lentil Soup

**Ingredients:**
- 1 cup green or brown lentils, rinsed and drained
- 1 small head of cabbage, thinly sliced
- 1 onion, diced
- 2 carrots, peeled and sliced
- 2 celery stalks, chopped
- 3 cloves garlic, minced
- 1 can (14 oz) diced tomatoes
- 6 cups vegetable broth
- 1 teaspoon ground cumin
- 1 teaspoon paprika
- Salt and pepper, to taste
- 2 tablespoons olive oil
- Fresh parsley, for garnish (optional)

**Instructions:**
1. **Sauté Vegetables:**
   - In a large pot, heat olive oil over medium heat. Add diced onion, sliced carrots, chopped celery, and minced garlic. Sauté until the vegetables are softened, about 5 minutes.
2. **Add Lentils and Spices:**
   - Stir in the lentils, ground cumin, paprika, salt, and pepper. Cook for an additional 2 minutes to toast the spices.

3. **Pour in Broth and Tomatoes:**
   - Pour in the vegetable broth and add the diced tomatoes (with their juice). Bring the mixture to a boil.
4. **Simmer:**
   - Reduce the heat to low, cover the pot, and let the soup simmer for 20-25 minutes or until the lentils are tender.
5. **Add Cabbage:**
   - Stir in the thinly sliced cabbage and cook for an additional 10-15 minutes or until the cabbage is tender.
6. **Adjust Seasoning:**
   - Taste the soup and adjust the seasoning, adding more salt and pepper if necessary.
7. **Serve:**
   - Ladle the soup into bowls and garnish with fresh parsley if desired.

**Benefits:**
1. **High in Fiber:** Lentils and cabbage are excellent sources of dietary fiber, promoting digestive health and helping with weight management.
2. **Rich in Vitamins and Minerals:** Cabbage provides vitamins like C and K, while lentils offer iron and folate.

3. **Low in Calories:** This soup is low in calories, making it a great option for those looking to maintain a healthy weight.
4. **Vegetarian Protein:** Lentils are a good source of plant-based protein, contributing to muscle health and overall satiety.
5. **Heart Health:** The combination of vegetables and lentils supports heart health by providing essential nutrients and promoting a balanced diet.

**Application:**
- **Lunch or Dinner:** Serve this hearty soup as a main course for a light and nutritious lunch or dinner.
- **Meal Prep:** Make a batch ahead of time for easy meal prep throughout the week, allowing the flavors to meld and intensify.
- **Side Dish:** Pair a smaller portion of the soup with a sandwich or salad for a well-rounded meal.

EAT TO BEAT YOUR DIET RECIPES BOOK

## Blackened Tilapia Tacos with Cabbage Slaw

**Ingredients:**
For the Blackened Tilapia:
- 4 tilapia fillets
- 1 tablespoon smoked paprika
- 1 teaspoon dried thyme
- 1 teaspoon onion powder
- 1 teaspoon garlic powder
- 1/2 teaspoon cayenne pepper
- Salt and pepper to taste
- 2 tablespoons olive oil

For the Cabbage Slaw:
- 2 cups shredded green cabbage
- 1/2 cup thinly sliced red onion
- 1/4 cup chopped fresh cilantro
- Juice of 1 lime
- 2 tablespoons plain Greek yogurt
- Salt and pepper to taste

For Assembling Tacos:
- 8 small corn or whole wheat tortillas
- Avocado slices (optional)
- Lime wedges for serving

**Instructions:**
**Blackened Tilapia:**
1. **Preheat Pan:**
    - In a small bowl, mix smoked paprika, dried thyme, onion powder, garlic powder, cayenne pepper, salt, and pepper. Rub the

spice mixture over both sides of each tilapia fillet.
2. **Cook Tilapia:**
    - Heat olive oil in a skillet over medium-high heat. Cook the tilapia fillets for 3-4 minutes per side or until the fish is cooked through and easily flaked with a fork.

**Cabbage Slaw:**
1. **Prepare Slaw:**
    - In a large bowl, combine shredded cabbage, sliced red onion, chopped cilantro, lime juice, Greek yogurt, salt, and pepper. Toss until well combined.
2. **Assemble Tacos:**
    - Warm the tortillas according to the package instructions. Place a blackened tilapia fillet on each tortilla.
3. **Add Slaw:**
    - Top each fillet with a generous portion of the cabbage slaw.
4. **Optional Toppings:**
    - Add avocado slices on top if desired.
5. **Serve:**
    - Serve the tacos with lime wedges on the side.

## EAT TO BEAT YOUR DIET RECIPES BOOK

**Benefits:**
1. **Lean Protein:** Tilapia is a low-fat, high-protein fish, contributing to muscle health and satiety.
2. **Heart-Healthy Spices:** The blackened seasoning includes spices like paprika and thyme, which may have heart-healthy benefits.
3. **Nutrient-Rich Cabbage:** Cabbage is a good source of vitamins C and K, as well as fiber, promoting digestive health.
4. **Probiotics from Yogurt:** Greek yogurt in the slaw provides probiotics, beneficial for gut health.

**Application:**
- **Quick Dinner Option:** These tacos are perfect for a quick and flavorful dinner option, especially for busy weeknights.
- **Entertaining:** Impress guests with a taco bar, allowing them to assemble their own tacos with a variety of toppings.
- **Healthy Lunch:** Pack the components separately and assemble the tacos just before eating for a fresh and satisfying lunch.

## Mango and Chicken Lettuce Wraps

**Ingredients:**
For the Chicken:
- 1 lb boneless, skinless chicken breast, thinly sliced
- 2 tablespoons soy sauce
- 1 tablespoon hoisin sauce
- 1 tablespoon sesame oil
- 1 teaspoon fresh ginger, minced
- 2 cloves garlic, minced
- 1 tablespoon olive oil

For the Mango Salsa:
- 1 ripe mango, peeled, pitted, and diced
- 1/2 red bell pepper, finely chopped
- 1/4 cup red onion, finely chopped
- 1/4 cup fresh cilantro, chopped
- Juice of 1 lime
- Salt and pepper to taste

For the Lettuce Wraps:
- Large lettuce leaves (such as butter or iceberg)

**Instructions:**
**Chicken:**
1. **Marinate Chicken:**
    - In a bowl, combine soy sauce, hoisin sauce, sesame oil, minced ginger, and minced garlic. Add sliced chicken and marinate for at least 15 minutes.

# EAT TO BEAT YOUR DIET RECIPES BOOK

2. **Cook Chicken:**
   - Heat olive oil in a skillet over medium-high heat. Add the marinated chicken and cook until fully cooked and slightly caramelized, about 5-7 minutes.

**Mango Salsa:**
1. **Prepare Salsa:**
   - In a separate bowl, combine diced mango, chopped red bell pepper, chopped red onion, cilantro, lime juice, salt, and pepper. Mix well.

**Assemble Lettuce Wraps:**
1. **Lay Out Lettuce Leaves:**
   - Arrange large lettuce leaves on a serving platter.
2. **Add Chicken:**
   - Place a spoonful of the cooked chicken in the center of each lettuce leaf.
3. **Top with Mango Salsa:**
   - Spoon the mango salsa over the chicken in each lettuce wrap.
4. **Serve:**
   - Serve the mango and chicken lettuce wraps immediately.

**Benefits:**
1. **Lean Protein:** Chicken breast provides a lean source of protein, essential for muscle health.

2. **Vitamins and Antioxidants:** Mango is rich in vitamins A and C, providing antioxidants that support immune health.
3. **Low-Calorie Option:** Lettuce wraps offer a lower-calorie alternative to traditional wraps or tacos.
4. **Flavorful Spices:** The combination of soy sauce, hoisin sauce, ginger, and garlic adds flavor without excess calories or sodium.

**Application:**
- **Light Lunch or Dinner:** Enjoy these lettuce wraps as a light and refreshing lunch or dinner option.
- **Appetizer:** Serve smaller portions as an appetizer at gatherings or parties.
- **Picnic or Outdoor Meal:** Pack the components separately for a portable and mess-free outdoor meal.

## Zucchini Noodles with Pesto and Cherry Tomatoes

**Ingredients:**
For the Zucchini Noodles:
- 4 medium zucchinis, spiralized into noodles
- 1 tablespoon olive oil
- Salt and pepper to taste

For the Pesto:
- 2 cups fresh basil leaves, packed
- 1/2 cup grated Parmesan cheese
- 1/2 cup pine nuts or walnuts
- 2 cloves garlic, minced
- 1/2 cup extra-virgin olive oil
- Salt and pepper to taste
- Juice of 1 lemon (optional)

For Topping:
- 1 cup cherry tomatoes, halved

**Instructions:**
**Zucchini Noodles:**
1. **Prepare Zucchini Noodles:**
   - Spiralize the zucchinis into noodle shapes. If you don't have a spiralizer, you can use a vegetable peeler to create long, thin strips.
2. **Sauté Zucchini:**
   - Heat olive oil in a large skillet over medium heat. Add the zucchini noodles and sauté for 2-3 minutes

until just tender. Season with salt and pepper.

**Pesto:**
1. **Combine Ingredients:**
   - In a food processor, combine basil, Parmesan cheese, pine nuts (or walnuts), and minced garlic.
2. **Blend:**
   - While the food processor is running, slowly drizzle in the olive oil until the pesto reaches your desired consistency. Add salt and pepper to taste. If you like, add lemon juice for a citrusy kick.

**Assemble:**
1. **Toss Zucchini with Pesto:**
   - In a large bowl, toss the sautéed zucchini noodles with the freshly made pesto until well coated.
2. **Top with Cherry Tomatoes:**
   - Add the halved cherry tomatoes on top of the zucchini noodles.
3. **Serve:**
   - Serve immediately, either warm or at room temperature.

**Benefits:**
1. **Low-Carb Option:** Zucchini noodles provide a low-carb alternative to traditional pasta.

## EAT TO BEAT YOUR DIET RECIPES BOOK

2. **Rich in Vitamins:** Zucchini is a good source of vitamins A and C, contributing to immune health.
3. **Healthy Fats:** Pesto made with olive oil, nuts, and Parmesan cheese provides heart-healthy fats.
4. **Antioxidants:** Basil and cherry tomatoes are rich in antioxidants that promote overall health.

**Application:**
- **Light Dinner Option:** Enjoy this dish as a light and flavorful dinner option.
- **Side Dish:** Serve as a refreshing side dish to complement grilled chicken, fish, or other protein sources.
- **Picnic or Potluck Dish:** This dish is great for picnics or potlucks as it can be served at room temperature.

## Kale and Quinoa Stuffed Bell Peppers

**Ingredients:**
For the Stuffed Bell Peppers:
- 4 large bell peppers, halved and seeds removed
- 1 cup quinoa, rinsed and cooked according to package instructions
- 2 cups kale, finely chopped
- 1 can (15 oz) black beans, drained and rinsed
- 1 cup cherry tomatoes, diced
- 1 cup feta cheese, crumbled (optional)
- 2 cloves garlic, minced
- 1 teaspoon cumin
- 1 teaspoon paprika
- Salt and pepper to taste
- Olive oil for drizzling

For the Avocado Cream Sauce:
- 2 ripe avocados, peeled and pitted
- 1/4 cup plain Greek yogurt
- Juice of 1 lime
- Salt and pepper to taste

**Instructions:**
**Stuffed Bell Peppers:**
1. **Preheat Oven:**
   - Preheat the oven to 375°F (190°C).
2. **Prepare Bell Peppers:**
   - Cut the bell peppers in half lengthwise and remove the seeds

and membranes. Place them in a baking dish.
3. **Cook Quinoa:**
   - Cook the quinoa according to the package instructions and set aside.
4. **Sauté Kale and Garlic:**
   - In a skillet, sauté the chopped kale and minced garlic in a drizzle of olive oil until the kale is wilted.
5. **Combine Ingredients:**
   - In a large bowl, combine the cooked quinoa, sautéed kale, black beans, cherry tomatoes, feta cheese (if using), cumin, paprika, salt, and pepper. Mix well.
6. **Stuff Bell Peppers:**
   - Stuff each bell pepper half with the quinoa mixture, pressing it down gently.
7. **Bake:**
   - Drizzle a little olive oil over the stuffed peppers. Cover the baking dish with foil and bake for 25-30 minutes or until the peppers are tender.

**Avocado Cream Sauce:**
1. **Prepare Sauce:**
   - In a blender or food processor, combine ripe avocados, Greek yogurt, lime juice, salt, and pepper. Blend until smooth.

# EAT TO BEAT YOUR DIET RECIPES BOOK

2. **Serve:**
   - Drizzle the stuffed bell peppers with avocado cream sauce before serving.

**Benefits:**
1. **Protein and Fiber:** Quinoa and black beans provide a combination of protein and fiber for a satisfying and nutritious meal.
2. **Vitamins and Antioxidants:** Kale and cherry tomatoes are rich in vitamins A and C, as well as antioxidants.
3. **Healthy Fats:** Avocado cream sauce adds healthy fats, contributing to a balanced and satiating dish.

**Application:**
- **Main Course:** Serve these stuffed bell peppers as a flavorful and nutritious main course.
- **Meal Prep:** These stuffed peppers are great for meal prep, providing a convenient and healthy option for lunches or dinners throughout the week.
- **Vegetarian Option:** Ideal for those seeking a hearty and delicious vegetarian or plant-based meal.

## Egg White Omelette with Spinach and Feta

**Ingredients:**
- 4 large egg whites
- 1 cup fresh spinach, chopped
- 1/4 cup crumbled feta cheese
- 1/4 cup cherry tomatoes, halved
- 1/4 cup red onion, finely chopped
- 1 clove garlic, minced
- 1 tablespoon olive oil
- Salt and pepper to taste
- Fresh herbs (such as parsley or chives) for garnish (optional)

**Instructions:**
1. **Prepare Vegetables:**
   - In a skillet, heat olive oil over medium heat. Add chopped spinach, cherry tomatoes, red onion, and minced garlic. Sauté for 2-3 minutes until the vegetables are slightly softened.
2. **Whisk Egg Whites:**
   - In a bowl, whisk the egg whites until frothy. Season with salt and pepper to taste.
3. **Add Egg Whites to Pan:**
   - Pour the whisked egg whites evenly over the sautéed vegetables in the skillet.

4. **Cook Omelette:**
    - Allow the eggs to set around the edges. As the edges firm up, gently lift them with a spatula to let the uncooked egg flow underneath.
5. **Add Feta Cheese:**
    - Sprinkle crumbled feta cheese over one half of the omelette.
6. **Fold and Serve:**
    - Once the egg whites are fully cooked, fold the omelette in half using the spatula. Slide it onto a plate.
7. **Garnish and Serve:**
    - Garnish with fresh herbs if desired. Serve immediately.

**Benefits:**
1. **Low-Calorie and High-Protein:** Egg whites are low in calories and high in protein, making them a nutritious and satiating option.
2. **Leafy Greens:** Spinach provides essential vitamins, minerals, and antioxidants while adding vibrant color to the dish.
3. **Healthy Fats:** Feta cheese adds a burst of flavor and healthy fats to the omelette.
4. **Vitamins from Tomatoes:** Cherry tomatoes contribute vitamins A and C, as well as antioxidants.

**Application:**
- **Breakfast or Brunch:** Enjoy this egg white omelette as a healthy and satisfying breakfast or brunch option.
- **Post-Workout Meal:** A protein-packed option for refueling after a workout.
- **Light Dinner:** Serve with a side salad for a light and nutritious dinner.

## Turkey and Vegetable Lettuce Wraps

**Ingredients:**
For the Turkey Mixture:
- 1 lb lean ground turkey
- 1 tablespoon olive oil
- 1 onion, finely chopped
- 2 cloves garlic, minced
- 1 red bell pepper, diced
- 1 zucchini, diced
- 1 carrot, shredded
- 2 tablespoons low-sodium soy sauce
- 1 tablespoon hoisin sauce
- 1 teaspoon fresh ginger, grated
- 1 teaspoon sesame oil
- Salt and pepper to taste
- Butter lettuce leaves for wrapping

For Garnish:
- Fresh cilantro, chopped
- Green onions, sliced
- Sesame seeds (optional)

**Instructions:**
1. **Sauté Turkey:**
    - In a large skillet, heat olive oil over medium-high heat. Add ground turkey and cook until browned and cooked through. Drain excess fat if necessary.

2. **Add Aromatics:**
    - Add chopped onion, minced garlic, and grated ginger to the skillet. Sauté until the onions are translucent.
3. **Vegetables:**
    - Add diced red bell pepper, zucchini, and shredded carrot to the skillet. Cook for 3-4 minutes until the vegetables are slightly tender.
4. **Sauce:**
    - Pour in low-sodium soy sauce, hoisin sauce, and sesame oil. Stir well to combine. Season with salt and pepper to taste.
5. **Simmer:**
    - Let the mixture simmer for an additional 2-3 minutes, allowing the flavors to meld.
6. **Assemble Lettuce Wraps:**
    - Spoon the turkey and vegetable mixture onto individual butter lettuce leaves.
7. **Garnish:**
    - Garnish with chopped fresh cilantro, sliced green onions, and sesame seeds if desired.

**Benefits:**
1. **Lean Protein:** Turkey is a lean source of protein, essential for muscle health and satiety.

2. **Colorful Vegetables:** Bell peppers, zucchini, and carrots provide a variety of vitamins, minerals, and antioxidants.
3. **Flavorful Sauces:** Low-sodium soy sauce and hoisin sauce add depth and flavor without excess sodium.
4. **Low-Carb Option:** Lettuce wraps offer a low-carb alternative to traditional wraps or tortillas.

**Application:**
- **Healthy Lunch or Dinner:** These lettuce wraps make for a light and healthy lunch or dinner option.
- **Appetizer:** Serve smaller portions as an appetizer for gatherings or parties.
- **Meal Prep:** Prepare the turkey and vegetable mixture ahead of time for quick and convenient meal prep throughout the week.

## Cauliflower Pizza with Veggie Toppings

**Ingredients:**
For the Cauliflower Pizza Crust:
- 1 medium cauliflower head, riced (about 4 cups)
- 1 cup shredded mozzarella cheese
- 1 large egg
- 1 teaspoon dried oregano
- 1 teaspoon garlic powder
- Salt and pepper to taste

For the Pizza Toppings:
- Tomato sauce (store-bought or homemade)
- 1 bell pepper, thinly sliced
- 1 red onion, thinly sliced
- 1 cup cherry tomatoes, halved
- 1 cup sliced mushrooms
- 1 cup baby spinach leaves
- 1 cup shredded mozzarella cheese
- Olive oil for drizzling
- Fresh basil or parsley for garnish (optional)

**Instructions:**
**Cauliflower Pizza Crust:**
1. **Prepare Cauliflower Rice:**
    - Remove the stem and leaves from the cauliflower head. Cut it into florets and pulse in a food processor until it resembles rice.

# EAT TO BEAT YOUR DIET RECIPES BOOK

2. **Steam and Drain:**
   - Steam the cauliflower rice in a microwave or on the stovetop until tender. Let it cool, then place it in a clean kitchen towel and squeeze out excess moisture.
3. **Mix Ingredients:**
   - In a bowl, combine the cauliflower rice, shredded mozzarella, egg, dried oregano, garlic powder, salt, and pepper. Mix until well combined.
4. **Form Crust:**
   - Press the cauliflower mixture onto a parchment-lined baking sheet, forming a thin, even crust.
5. **Bake:**
   - Bake the crust in a preheated oven at 425°F (220°C) for 15-20 minutes or until golden brown.

**Assemble and Bake Pizza:**
1. **Prep Toppings:**
   - While the crust is baking, prepare your favorite pizza toppings. Slice the bell pepper, red onion, cherry tomatoes, mushrooms, and gather the baby spinach.
2. **Add Sauce and Toppings:**
   - Once the crust is golden, spread tomato sauce over the crust, leaving a border around the edges.

Sprinkle shredded mozzarella cheese evenly, then arrange the sliced vegetables on top.
3. **Bake Again:**
   - Return the pizza to the oven and bake for an additional 10-15 minutes or until the cheese is melted and bubbly.
4. **Garnish and Serve:**
   - Drizzle the pizza with olive oil and garnish with fresh basil or parsley if desired. Slice and serve.

**Benefits:**
1. **Low-Carb Alternative:** Cauliflower crust is a nutritious and low-carb substitute for traditional pizza dough.
2. **Vegetable-Packed:** The veggie toppings provide essential vitamins, minerals, and antioxidants.
3. **Gluten-Free:** This pizza is naturally gluten-free, making it suitable for those with gluten sensitivities.

**Application:**
- **Healthy Pizza Night:** Enjoy this cauliflower pizza as a healthier alternative to traditional pizza for a fun and nutritious pizza night.
- **Family-Friendly Meal:** Get the family involved by letting everyone choose their favorite toppings for a customized pizza experience.

## EAT TO BEAT YOUR DIET RECIPES BOOK

- **Entertaining:** Serve as a unique and delicious appetizer or main course for gatherings or parties.

## Greek Yogurt Parfait with Fresh Berries

**Ingredients:**
- 2 cups Greek yogurt (unsweetened)
- 1 cup mixed fresh berries (strawberries, blueberries, raspberries)
- 1/2 cup granola
- 2 tablespoons honey or maple syrup
- 1/4 cup chopped nuts (such as almonds or walnuts)
- Fresh mint leaves for garnish (optional)

**Instructions:**
1. **Layer Greek Yogurt:**
   - In serving glasses or bowls, start by adding a layer of Greek yogurt.
2. **Add Berries:**
   - Add a layer of mixed fresh berries on top of the Greek yogurt.
3. **Sprinkle Granola:**
   - Sprinkle a layer of granola over the berries. This adds crunch and texture.
4. **Repeat Layers:**
   - Repeat the layers until you reach the top of the glass or bowl, finishing with a layer of berries.
5. **Drizzle with Honey:**
   - Drizzle honey or maple syrup over the top for added sweetness.

# EAT TO BEAT YOUR DIET RECIPES BOOK

6. **Top with Nuts:**
   - Sprinkle chopped nuts over the parfait for a boost of healthy fats and extra crunch.
7. **Garnish:**
   - Garnish with fresh mint leaves for a burst of freshness (optional).
8. **Serve Immediately:**
   - Serve the Greek Yogurt Parfait immediately to enjoy the contrast of creamy yogurt, juicy berries, and crunchy granola.

**Benefits:**
1. **Protein-Rich:** Greek yogurt is a excellent source of protein, aiding in muscle repair and satiety.
2. **Antioxidant-Rich Berries:** Fresh berries provide a variety of antioxidants, vitamins, and minerals for overall health.
3. **Whole Grains from Granola:** Granola adds whole grains, fiber, and energy-boosting nutrients to the parfait.
4. **Healthy Fats from Nuts:** Chopped nuts contribute healthy fats, adding richness and satiety.

**Application:**
- **Breakfast or Snack:** Enjoy this parfait as a wholesome and filling breakfast or a satisfying snack.

- **Dessert Alternative:** Serve as a healthier dessert option for those who enjoy a sweet treat without excess sugar.
- **Brunch or Party Dish:** Prepare individual parfaits for brunch gatherings or as a colorful addition to a party spread.

EAT TO BEAT YOUR DIET RECIPES BOOK

## Recipe: Spaghetti Squash with Turkey Bolognese

**Ingredients:**
For the Spaghetti Squash:
- 1 medium-sized spaghetti squash
- Olive oil
- Salt and pepper

For the Turkey Bolognese:
- 1 lb lean ground turkey
- 1 tablespoon olive oil
- 1 onion, finely chopped
- 2 cloves garlic, minced
- 1 carrot, grated
- 1 celery stalk, finely chopped
- 1 can (14 oz) crushed tomatoes
- 1/2 cup tomato sauce
- 1 teaspoon dried oregano
- 1 teaspoon dried basil
- Salt and pepper to taste
- Fresh basil or parsley for garnish
- Grated Parmesan cheese for serving (optional)

**Instructions:**
**Spaghetti Squash:**
1. **Preheat Oven:**
   - Preheat the oven to 400°F (200°C).
2. **Prepare Squash:**
   - Cut the spaghetti squash in half lengthwise. Scoop out the seeds.

3. **Season and Roast:**
    - Drizzle the cut sides of the squash with olive oil and sprinkle with salt and pepper. Place them cut side down on a baking sheet. Roast in the preheated oven for 40-45 minutes or until the flesh is tender.
4. **Scrape and Fluff:**
    - Using a fork, scrape the strands of spaghetti squash away from the skin. Fluff the strands to create a spaghetti-like texture.

**Turkey Bolognese:**
1. **Cook Turkey:**
    - In a large skillet, heat olive oil over medium-high heat. Add ground turkey and cook until browned, breaking it up with a spoon as it cooks.
2. **Sauté Vegetables:**
    - Add chopped onion, minced garlic, grated carrot, and chopped celery to the skillet. Sauté until the vegetables are softened.
3. **Add Tomatoes and Sauce:**
    - Pour in crushed tomatoes and tomato sauce. Stir to combine.
4. **Season:**
    - Add dried oregano, dried basil, salt, and pepper. Stir well and let the

sauce simmer for 15-20 minutes, allowing the flavors to meld.
5. **Serve:**
    - Spoon the turkey bolognese over the roasted spaghetti squash. Garnish with fresh basil or parsley and Parmesan cheese if desired.

**Benefits:**
1. **Lean Protein:** Turkey provides a lean source of protein, essential for muscle health.
2. **Vegetable Rich:** The bolognese sauce is packed with vegetables like onions, carrots, and celery, offering a variety of nutrients.
3. **Low-Carb Option:** Spaghetti squash is a low-carb alternative to traditional pasta, suitable for those watching their carbohydrate intake.

**Application:**
- **Healthy Dinner Option:** Enjoy this dish as a nutritious and satisfying dinner option.
- **Meal Prep:** Prepare the turkey bolognese in advance for easy meal prep throughout the week.
- **Family-Friendly Meal:** A crowd-pleaser that's suitable for the whole family.

## Vegetarian Stir-Fry with Tofu and Broccoli

**Ingredients:**
For the Stir-Fry Sauce:
- 1/4 cup soy sauce
- 2 tablespoons hoisin sauce
- 1 tablespoon rice vinegar
- 1 tablespoon sesame oil
- 1 tablespoon maple syrup or honey
- 1 teaspoon cornstarch
- 1/2 cup vegetable broth

For the Stir-Fry:
- 14 oz (400g) extra-firm tofu, pressed and cubed
- 2 tablespoons soy sauce
- 1 tablespoon sesame oil
- 1 tablespoon vegetable oil
- 3 cups broccoli florets
- 1 red bell pepper, thinly sliced
- 1 carrot, julienned
- 3 cloves garlic, minced
- 1 tablespoon fresh ginger, grated
- Cooked brown rice or quinoa for serving
- Sesame seeds and chopped green onions for garnish

**Instructions:**
**Stir-Fry Sauce:**
1. **Mix Ingredients:**
    - In a bowl, whisk together soy sauce, hoisin sauce, rice vinegar, sesame

oil, maple syrup (or honey), cornstarch, and vegetable broth. Set aside.

**Tofu:**
1. **Press Tofu:**
   - Press the tofu to remove excess water. Cut the pressed tofu into cubes and marinate with soy sauce for at least 15 minutes.
2. **Cook Tofu:**
   - In a large skillet or wok, heat sesame oil and vegetable oil over medium-high heat. Add the marinated tofu cubes and cook until golden brown on all sides. Remove from the skillet and set aside.

**Vegetarian Stir-Fry:**
1. **Sauté Vegetables:**
   - In the same skillet, add a bit more oil if needed. Sauté garlic and ginger until fragrant. Add broccoli, bell pepper, and carrot. Stir-fry for 3-4 minutes until the vegetables are crisp-tender.
2. **Combine Tofu and Sauce:**
   - Add the cooked tofu back to the skillet with the vegetables. Pour the prepared stir-fry sauce over the tofu and vegetables. Toss everything together to coat evenly.

3. **Simmer:**
   - Allow the mixture to simmer for an additional 2-3 minutes, allowing the sauce to thicken.
4. **Serve:**
   - Serve the vegetarian stir-fry over cooked brown rice or quinoa. Garnish with sesame seeds and chopped green onions.

**Benefits:**
1. **Protein-Rich Tofu:** Tofu serves as a plant-based protein source, essential for a vegetarian diet.
2. **Nutrient-Dense Vegetables:** Broccoli, bell pepper, and carrots provide a variety of vitamins, minerals, and antioxidants.
3. **Healthy Fats:** Sesame oil adds a rich flavor and healthy fats to the stir-fry.
4. **Wholesome Carbohydrates:** Brown rice or quinoa adds complex carbohydrates for sustained energy.

**Application:**
- **Quick Weeknight Meal:** This stir-fry is perfect for a quick and easy weeknight dinner.
- **Meal Prep:** Make a batch and portion it for convenient and nutritious meal prep throughout the week.
- **Customizable:** Feel free to customize the vegetables based on what's in season or what you have on hand.

## Quinoa Salad with Mixed Vegetables and Lemon Vinaigrette

**Ingredients:**
For the Quinoa Salad:
- 1 cup quinoa, rinsed
- 2 cups water or vegetable broth
- 1 cup cherry tomatoes, halved
- 1 cucumber, diced
- 1 bell pepper (any color), diced
- 1/2 red onion, finely chopped
- 1/4 cup Kalamata olives, pitted and sliced
- 1/4 cup feta cheese, crumbled (optional)
- Fresh parsley or basil, chopped for garnish

For the Lemon Vinaigrette:
- 1/4 cup extra-virgin olive oil
- Zest and juice of 1 lemon
- 1 tablespoon Dijon mustard
- 1 clove garlic, minced
- Salt and pepper to taste

**Instructions:**
**Quinoa:**
1. **Cook Quinoa:**
    - In a medium saucepan, combine quinoa and water (or vegetable broth). Bring to a boil, then reduce heat to low, cover, and simmer for 15 minutes or until quinoa is cooked and water is absorbed. Fluff with a fork and let it cool.

**Lemon Vinaigrette:**
1. **Whisk Ingredients:**
   - In a small bowl, whisk together olive oil, lemon zest, lemon juice, Dijon mustard, minced garlic, salt, and pepper. Set aside.

**Quinoa Salad:**
1. **Combine Ingredients:**
   - In a large bowl, combine cooked and cooled quinoa with cherry tomatoes, cucumber, bell pepper, red onion, Kalamata olives, and feta cheese if using.
2. **Add Lemon Vinaigrette:**
   - Pour the lemon vinaigrette over the quinoa and vegetables. Toss gently to coat everything evenly.
3. **Garnish:**
   - Garnish the quinoa salad with chopped fresh parsley or basil.
4. **Chill and Serve:**
   - Refrigerate the salad for at least 30 minutes to allow the flavors to meld. Serve chilled.

**Benefits:**
1. **Complete Protein:** Quinoa is a complete protein, providing all essential amino acids.
2. **Nutrient-Rich Vegetables:** The mixed vegetables contribute a variety of vitamins, minerals, and antioxidants.

# EAT TO BEAT YOUR DIET RECIPES BOOK

3. **Healthy Fats:** Olive oil in the vinaigrette adds heart-healthy monounsaturated fats.
4. **Refreshing and Light:** Lemon vinaigrette adds a refreshing and light flavor to the salad.

**Application:**
- **Lunch or Dinner Option:** Enjoy this quinoa salad as a light and satisfying lunch or dinner.
- **Potluck or Picnic Dish:** Bring this colorful and flavorful salad to potlucks, picnics, or barbecues.
- **Meal Prep:** Prepare a batch for meal prep, dividing it into individual containers for convenient and healthy lunches throughout the week.

## Chickpea and Spinach Curry

**Ingredients:**
- 2 cans (15 oz each) chickpeas, drained and rinsed
- 2 tablespoons vegetable oil
- 1 large onion, finely chopped
- 3 cloves garlic, minced
- 1 tablespoon fresh ginger, grated
- 1 teaspoon ground cumin
- 1 teaspoon ground coriander
- 1 teaspoon turmeric
- 1 teaspoon curry powder
- 1/2 teaspoon cayenne pepper (adjust to taste)
- 1 can (14 oz) diced tomatoes
- 1 can (14 oz) coconut milk
- 4 cups fresh spinach, washed and chopped
- Salt and pepper to taste
- Fresh cilantro, chopped, for garnish
- Cooked basmati rice or naan for serving

**Instructions:**
1. **Sauté Aromatics:**
   - In a large skillet or pot, heat vegetable oil over medium heat. Add chopped onions and sauté until they become translucent.
2. **Add Garlic and Ginger:**
   - Add minced garlic and grated ginger to the onions. Sauté for an

additional 1-2 minutes until fragrant.
3. **Spices:**
   - Add ground cumin, ground coriander, turmeric, curry powder, and cayenne pepper to the skillet. Stir well to coat the aromatics with the spices.
4. **Chickpeas:**
   - Incorporate the drained and rinsed chickpeas into the spice mixture. Stir to coat the chickpeas evenly.
5. **Tomatoes:**
   - Pour in the diced tomatoes (with their juices) and mix well. Allow the mixture to simmer for 5-7 minutes.
6. **Coconut Milk:**
   - Stir in the coconut milk, bringing the curry to a gentle simmer. Let it cook for an additional 10-15 minutes, allowing the flavors to meld.
7. **Add Spinach:**
   - Add the chopped spinach to the curry. Cook until the spinach wilts and becomes tender.
8. **Season:**
   - Season the curry with salt and pepper to taste. Adjust the spices if needed.

9. **Serve:**
    - Serve the Chickpea and Spinach Curry over cooked basmati rice or with warm naan. Garnish with chopped cilantro.

**Benefits:**
1. **Plant-Based Protein:** Chickpeas are a rich source of plant-based protein, making this curry a nutritious option for vegetarians and vegans.
2. **Leafy Greens:** Spinach adds a dose of iron, vitamins, and antioxidants to the dish.
3. **Healthy Fats:** Coconut milk provides healthy fats, contributing to a creamy and satisfying texture.
4. **Anti-Inflammatory Spices:** The combination of cumin, coriander, turmeric, and curry powder not only enhances flavor but also offers potential anti-inflammatory benefits.

**Application:**
- **Weeknight Dinner:** This quick and easy recipe is perfect for a flavorful weeknight dinner.
- **Meal Prep:** Make a batch for meal prep and enjoy delicious lunches throughout the week.
- **Entertaining:** Impress guests with a hearty and flavorful chickpea and spinach curry at your next gathering.

## Salmon and Asparagus Foil Packets

**Ingredients:**
- 4 salmon fillets (6 oz each)
- 1 bunch asparagus, tough ends trimmed
- 1 lemon, thinly sliced
- 4 cloves garlic, minced
- 2 tablespoons fresh dill, chopped
- 2 tablespoons olive oil
- Salt and pepper to taste
- 1 teaspoon smoked paprika (optional)
- Aluminum foil

**Instructions:**
1. **Preheat Oven:**
   - Preheat your oven to 400°F (200°C).
2. **Prepare Foil Packets:**
   - Tear off four large pieces of aluminum foil. Place a salmon fillet in the center of each piece of foil.
3. **Season Salmon:**
   - Season each salmon fillet with salt, pepper, and smoked paprika if using. Drizzle with olive oil and rub minced garlic on top.
4. **Assemble with Asparagus:**
   - Arrange a handful of asparagus spears alongside each salmon fillet. Place a couple of lemon slices on top

of the salmon, and sprinkle with fresh dill.
5. **Seal Foil Packets:**
   - Seal the foil packets tightly, ensuring that the edges are well-crimped to keep the steam inside during cooking.
6. **Bake:**
   - Place the foil packets on a baking sheet and bake in the preheated oven for 15-20 minutes, or until the salmon is cooked through and flakes easily with a fork.
7. **Serve:**
   - Carefully open the foil packets, being cautious of the hot steam. Serve the salmon and asparagus over a bed of rice, quinoa, or your preferred grain.

**Benefits:**
1. **Omega-3 Fatty Acids:** Salmon is rich in omega-3 fatty acids, which are essential for heart health and brain function.
2. **Lean Protein:** Salmon provides a high-quality, lean source of protein, important for muscle health.
3. **Antioxidant-Rich Asparagus:** Asparagus is loaded with antioxidants, vitamins, and minerals that contribute to overall health.

4. **Garlic and Dill for Flavor:** Garlic adds depth of flavor while dill provides a refreshing herbal note to the dish.

**Application:**
- **Quick Weeknight Dinner:** These foil packets make for a quick and easy weeknight dinner that requires minimal cleanup.
- **Outdoor Grilling:** Take the foil packets to the grill for a delicious outdoor cooking experience.
- **Meal Prep:** Prepare multiple foil packets in advance and refrigerate them until ready to bake for convenient meal prep.

## Turkey and Vegetable Skewers with Greek Yogurt Sauce

**Ingredients:**
For the Turkey and Vegetable Skewers:
- 1 lb lean ground turkey
- 1 red bell pepper, cut into chunks
- 1 zucchini, sliced into rounds
- 1 red onion, cut into wedges
- Cherry tomatoes
- 2 tablespoons olive oil
- 1 teaspoon dried oregano
- 1 teaspoon ground cumin
- 1 teaspoon smoked paprika
- Salt and pepper to taste
- Wooden skewers, soaked in water for at least 30 minutes

For the Greek Yogurt Sauce:
- 1 cup Greek yogurt
- 1 cucumber, grated and drained
- 2 cloves garlic, minced
- 1 tablespoon fresh dill, chopped
- 1 tablespoon lemon juice
- Salt and pepper to taste

**Instructions:**
**Turkey and Vegetable Skewers:**
1. **Preheat Grill:**
    - Preheat your grill or grill pan over medium-high heat.

# EAT TO BEAT YOUR DIET RECIPES BOOK

2. **Prepare Turkey Mixture:**
   - In a bowl, combine ground turkey with olive oil, dried oregano, ground cumin, smoked paprika, salt, and pepper. Mix well.
3. **Assemble Skewers:**
   - Thread the seasoned ground turkey onto the soaked wooden skewers, alternating with chunks of red bell pepper, zucchini slices, red onion wedges, and cherry tomatoes.
4. **Grill:**
   - Place the skewers on the preheated grill and cook for about 12-15 minutes, turning occasionally, until the turkey is cooked through and the vegetables are charred and tender.
5. **Greek Yogurt Sauce:**
   - While the skewers are grilling, prepare the Greek Yogurt Sauce. In a bowl, combine Greek yogurt, grated cucumber, minced garlic, chopped fresh dill, lemon juice, salt, and pepper. Mix well.
6. **Serve:**
   - Serve the Turkey and Vegetable Skewers with a generous drizzle of the Greek Yogurt Sauce on the side.

**Benefits:**
1. **Lean Protein:** Turkey is a lean source of protein, crucial for muscle health and satiety.
2. **Colorful Vegetables:** Bell peppers, zucchini, red onions, and cherry tomatoes provide a variety of vitamins, minerals, and antioxidants.
3. **Healthy Fats:** Olive oil and Greek yogurt contribute healthy fats to the dish.
4. **Probiotics from Greek Yogurt:** Greek yogurt in the sauce provides probiotics for gut health.

**Application:**
- **Outdoor Grilling:** These skewers are perfect for outdoor grilling, whether it's a family barbecue or a summer gathering.
- **Weeknight Dinner:** Prepare these skewers for a quick and flavorful weeknight dinner that's both healthy and delicious.
- **Entertaining:** Impress your guests with a visually appealing and tasty dish at your next gathering.

EAT TO BEAT YOUR DIET RECIPES BOOK

## Shrimp and Avocado Salad

**Ingredients:**
For the Salad:
- 1 lb large shrimp, peeled and deveined
- 2 avocados, diced
- 1 cup cherry tomatoes, halved
- 1 cucumber, sliced
- 1/4 red onion, thinly sliced
- 1/4 cup fresh cilantro, chopped
- Mixed salad greens (e.g., arugula, spinach, or mixed greens)

For the Dressing:
- 3 tablespoons olive oil
- 2 tablespoons fresh lime juice
- 1 teaspoon honey or maple syrup
- 1 clove garlic, minced
- Salt and pepper to taste

**Instructions:**
**Prepare Shrimp:**
1. **Cook Shrimp:**
    - In a large skillet, heat olive oil over medium-high heat. Add shrimp and cook for 2-3 minutes per side or until they turn pink and opaque. Remove from heat and set aside.

**Assemble Salad:**
1. **Combine Ingredients:**
    - In a large bowl, combine cooked shrimp, diced avocados, cherry tomatoes, sliced cucumber, red onion, and chopped cilantro.

2. **Add Salad Greens:**
    - Add a generous handful of mixed salad greens to the bowl.

**Prepare Dressing:**
1. **Whisk Ingredients:**
    - In a small bowl, whisk together olive oil, fresh lime juice, honey (or maple syrup), minced garlic, salt, and pepper.
2. **Drizzle Dressing:**
    - Drizzle the dressing over the salad and gently toss everything together until well combined.
3. **Serve:**
    - Divide the Shrimp and Avocado Salad among plates. Optionally, garnish with additional cilantro and lime wedges.

**Benefits:**
1. **Lean Protein:** Shrimp is a low-calorie, high-protein seafood option, aiding in muscle repair and satiety.
2. **Healthy Fats:** Avocados contribute heart-healthy monounsaturated fats, providing a creamy texture to the salad.
3. **Vitamins and Antioxidants:** Tomatoes, cucumbers, and salad greens offer a range of vitamins, minerals, and antioxidants.

4. **Light and Refreshing:** The lime-based dressing adds a refreshing and tangy flavor to the salad.

**Application:**
- **Lunch or Dinner Option:** Enjoy this Shrimp and Avocado Salad as a light and satisfying lunch or dinner.
- **Summer Entertaining:** Serve this vibrant salad at summer gatherings or picnics for a refreshing dish that's sure to impress.
- **Meal Prep:** Prepare the components in advance and assemble the salad for quick and convenient meal prep.

## Baked Cod with Lemon and Dill

**Ingredients:**
- 4 cod fillets (about 6 oz each)
- 2 tablespoons olive oil
- 2 tablespoons fresh lemon juice
- 2 cloves garlic, minced
- 1 tablespoon fresh dill, chopped
- Zest of one lemon
- Salt and pepper to taste
- Lemon slices for garnish
- Fresh dill for garnish

**Instructions:**
1. **Preheat Oven:**
   - Preheat your oven to 400°F (200°C).
2. **Prepare Cod:**
   - Pat the cod fillets dry with paper towels. Place them in a baking dish, leaving some space between each fillet.
3. **Make Marinade:**
   - In a small bowl, whisk together olive oil, fresh lemon juice, minced garlic, chopped fresh dill, lemon zest, salt, and pepper.
4. **Marinate Cod:**
   - Pour the marinade over the cod fillets, ensuring they are evenly

coated. Allow the cod to marinate for 15-20 minutes.
5. **Bake:**
   - Bake the cod in the preheated oven for 12-15 minutes or until the fish is opaque and easily flakes with a fork.
6. **Garnish:**
   - Garnish the baked cod with additional fresh dill and lemon slices.
7. **Serve:**
   - Serve the Baked Cod with Lemon and Dill over a bed of steamed vegetables, quinoa, or your favorite side dish.

**Benefits:**
1. **Lean Protein:** Cod is a lean source of protein, essential for muscle health and overall well-being.
2. **Heart-Healthy Fats:** Olive oil provides healthy monounsaturated fats, contributing to heart health.
3. **Vitamin C:** Fresh lemon juice adds a burst of vitamin C, known for its immune-boosting properties.
4. **Anti-Inflammatory:** Garlic and dill not only enhance flavor but also offer potential anti-inflammatory benefits.

# EAT TO BEAT YOUR DIET RECIPES BOOK

**Application:**
- **Weeknight Dinner:** This quick and easy recipe is perfect for a flavorful weeknight dinner.
- **Entertaining:** Impress guests with an elegant yet straightforward dish at your next dinner gathering.
- **Light and Healthy Option:** Serve as a light and healthy option for those looking for a delicious meal without excess calories.

## Sweet Potato and Black Bean Enchiladas

**Ingredients:**
For the Filling:
- 2 medium sweet potatoes, peeled and diced
- 1 can (15 oz) black beans, drained and rinsed
- 1 red bell pepper, diced
- 1 small red onion, finely chopped
- 2 cloves garlic, minced
- 1 teaspoon ground cumin
- 1 teaspoon chili powder
- Salt and pepper to taste
- 2 tablespoons olive oil

For the Enchilada Sauce:
- 1 can (15 oz) tomato sauce
- 1/2 cup vegetable broth
- 1 teaspoon ground cumin
- 1 teaspoon chili powder
- 1/2 teaspoon garlic powder
- Salt and pepper to taste

For Assembly:
- 8 whole wheat or corn tortillas
- 1 cup shredded Mexican cheese blend
- Fresh cilantro, chopped, for garnish
- Avocado slices, for serving (optional)
- Greek yogurt or sour cream, for serving (optional)

## Instructions:
### Filling:
1. **Roast Sweet Potatoes:**
   - Preheat the oven to 400°F (200°C). Toss the diced sweet potatoes with 1 tablespoon of olive oil, cumin, chili powder, salt, and pepper. Roast in the oven for 20-25 minutes or until tender.
2. **Sauté Vegetables:**
   - In a skillet, heat the remaining tablespoon of olive oil over medium heat. Sauté red bell pepper, red onion, and garlic until softened. Add black beans and roasted sweet potatoes. Stir to combine and cook for an additional 2-3 minutes. Set aside.

### Enchilada Sauce:
1. **Prepare Sauce:**
   - In a saucepan, combine tomato sauce, vegetable broth, cumin, chili powder, garlic powder, salt, and pepper. Bring to a simmer and cook for 5-7 minutes. Set aside.

### Assembly:
1. **Preheat Oven:**
   - Preheat the oven to 375°F (190°C).
2. **Assemble Enchiladas:**
   - In each tortilla, spoon a generous portion of the sweet potato and

# EAT TO BEAT YOUR DIET RECIPES BOOK

   black bean filling. Roll the tortillas and place them seam-side down in a baking dish.
3. **Pour Sauce:**
   - Pour the enchilada sauce over the rolled tortillas, making sure they are well-covered.
4. **Add Cheese:**
   - Sprinkle shredded Mexican cheese blend over the top of the enchiladas.
5. **Bake:**
   - Bake in the preheated oven for 20-25 minutes or until the cheese is melted and bubbly.
6. **Garnish and Serve:**
   - Remove from the oven and let it cool slightly. Garnish with chopped cilantro. Serve with avocado slices, Greek yogurt, or sour cream if desired.

**Benefits:**
1. **Nutrient-Rich Sweet Potatoes:** Sweet potatoes are high in fiber, vitamins, and antioxidants.
2. **Protein-Packed Black Beans:** Black beans provide a good source of plant-based protein and fiber.
3. **Vitamins and Minerals:** Bell peppers and onions contribute additional vitamins and minerals to the dish.

4. **Whole Grains:** Whole wheat or corn tortillas offer whole grains for sustained energy.

**Application:**
- **Meatless Monday Dinner:** This vegetarian dish is perfect for a Meatless Monday dinner.
- **Meal Prep:** Prepare a batch for meal prep, as enchiladas are easy to reheat for quick and satisfying lunches.
- **Family-Friendly:** A crowd-pleaser suitable for family dinners or gatherings.

## Grilled Chicken Breast with Herb Marinade

**Ingredients:**
For the Herb Marinade:
- 4 boneless, skinless chicken breasts
- 3 tablespoons olive oil
- 2 tablespoons fresh lemon juice
- 2 cloves garlic, minced
- 2 tablespoons fresh parsley, chopped
- 1 tablespoon fresh thyme leaves
- 1 tablespoon fresh rosemary, chopped
- Salt and pepper to taste

For Garnish:
- Fresh lemon wedges
- Fresh herbs for sprinkling (parsley, thyme, rosemary)

**Instructions:**
**Marinade:**
1. **Prepare Marinade:**
   - In a bowl, whisk together olive oil, fresh lemon juice, minced garlic, chopped parsley, thyme leaves, rosemary, salt, and pepper.
2. **Marinate Chicken:**
   - Place the chicken breasts in a resealable plastic bag or a shallow dish. Pour the herb marinade over the chicken, making sure each breast is well-coated. Seal the bag or cover the dish and refrigerate for

at least 30 minutes, or ideally, marinate for up to 4 hours.

**Grilling:**
1. **Preheat Grill:**
   - Preheat your grill to medium-high heat.
2. **Remove Chicken from Marinade:**
   - Remove the chicken from the refrigerator and let it come to room temperature for about 15 minutes.
3. **Grill Chicken:**
   - Grill the chicken breasts for 6-8 minutes per side or until they reach an internal temperature of 165°F (74°C) and the juices run clear. Cooking times may vary depending on the thickness of the chicken breasts.
4. **Rest and Garnish:**
   - Remove the chicken from the grill and let it rest for a few minutes. Garnish with fresh lemon wedges and sprinkle with additional fresh herbs.
5. **Serve:**
   - Serve the Grilled Chicken Breast with Herb Marinade alongside your favorite side dishes.

**Benefits:**
1. **Lean Protein:** Chicken breast is a lean source of protein, essential for muscle health and satiety.
2. **Heart-Healthy Fats:** Olive oil in the marinade provides heart-healthy monounsaturated fats.
3. **Antioxidant-Rich Herbs:** Fresh herbs like parsley, thyme, and rosemary not only add flavor but also contribute antioxidants and other health benefits.
4. **Low-Calorie Option:** Grilling keeps the chicken light and flavorful without excess calories.

**Application:**
- **Weeknight Dinner:** This quick and flavorful recipe is perfect for a simple weeknight dinner.
- **Summer BBQ:** Ideal for grilling at summer barbecues or gatherings.
- **Meal Prep:** Prepare a batch of grilled chicken to use in salads, wraps, or sandwiches for convenient and healthy meal prep.

## CONCLUSION

We sincerely hope that, as we approach the last pages of the "Eat to Beat Your Diet Recipes Book," you've discovered happiness, inspiration, and a fresh sense of empowerment in your pursuit of a more vibrant, healthy life.

This recipe collection is about more than just losing weight; it's about living a lifestyle that honors the significant relationship that exists between healthful, flavorful food and your general well-being.

We've learned about the benefits of enjoying each bite, the skill of mindful eating, and the nutritional value of a variety of ingredients during this culinary adventure. Every recipe has been created with the goal of enhancing the effectiveness and enjoyment of your weight loss journey.

Recall that this book serves as a tool—a guide—to assist you in navigating the frequently challenging realm of weight management and nutrition. The recipes in these pages are designed to tantalize your taste senses with a symphony of flavors and provide your body with the nutrients it needs.

# EAT TO BEAT YOUR DIET RECIPES BOOK

We want you to personalize each meal as you move from these recipes into your own kitchen. Try different flavors, enjoy what's in season, and take pleasure in cooking healthful meals. This is an invitation to explore, adjust, and enjoy the experience rather than a strict set of guidelines.

However, the adventure is far from over. As you continue on your journey to a better lifestyle, we hope that this book will be a reliable guide. Recall that every decision you make as you delve deeper into the world of nutrition is a step toward your overall health and wellbeing.

We are grateful that you let us share in your adventure. I hope you have colorful meals, happy moods, and unrelenting dedication to being a healthier version of yourself. Cheers to a life full of wholesome meals, delectable discoveries, and constant pursuit of your happiest, healthiest self.

Eat healthily, enjoy the trip, and use each delicious bite to help you beat your diet.

Cheers to you and your wellness journey!

Made in the USA
Monee, IL
02 January 2024